MORNING WEIGHT LOSS

3-Week Productivity Boosting Program To Help

You Get More Done And Shed Pounds,

Permanently!

John Mayo

A Note To My Loyal Reader:

As you are probably already aware from my other books, I put all 100% of my effort into every single book that I write. When I have a book on the go it's all I can think about because I want to deliver my readers with the best information that I possibly can. This is why I ask that if you enjoy this book, **please take the time to give it an honest review.** I would really appreciate it and so would other readers who are trying to sift through the nonsense books on Amazon and find the books worth buying. There are just so many people out there now trying to make a quick buck by selling worthless, lackluster books. While I don't deny that publishing books is my primary source of income, I take pride in the fact that my books are completely original and a product of my hard work and ever growing knowledge about fitness.

Thank you in advance,

- John Mayo

Table of Contents:

Chapter 1: Introduction

Wouldn't it be amazing if everyone could be a morning person? Imagine if you no longer had to dread the sound of your alarm clock and stumble angrily into the kitchen to make yourself a coffee to fuel you for long enough to make it to the shower. What if mornings didn't have to be such a struggle? Well, I'm here to tell you that it doesn't have to be a struggle at all, in fact, I can help you supercharge your morning routine so that your productivity can be boosted during the rest of your day. Wouldn't you love to lower your stress level first thing in the morning by only doing a small amount of reading an a short and simple 10-15 minute workout You may be shaking your head right now, telling yourself that it's not possible for you to become a morning person because you are just a complete mess when your alarm clock goes off. I was never a morning person either, but now I jump out of bed and attack my days with a ton of energy. I used to struggle to keep my eyes open first thing in the morning, but now I'm wide eyed and ready to go every single morning. What's the secret you ask? I'm going to tell you throughout this concise and informative book. I hate spending unnecessary money, and as much as you might not think that buying coffee adds up over time, it really does! Not to mention, the crash from coffee can be enough to throw you into an unwanted midday nap.

If you've read some of my other books then you're probably familiar with my writing style and who I am. If not, then I will be brief. I am a fitness fanatic, an ex competitive kayaker, current fitness/kayaking coach and my goal is to better the lives of others by transferring my knowledge via eBooks and personal online coaching. I honestly believe that many of today's psychological disorders can be attributed to a lack of health and fitness. I also believe that living a healthy life is way easier than people make it out to be. Obviously it requires sacrifice and determination, but if you put your mind to it you can achieve any of your fitness goals.

The benefits of being a morning person are innumerable. If you have a supercharged morning routine you will feel better physically and psychologically, you will have a clear mind, get more done throughout the day, feel less fatigued as the day progresses, be less moody during the day and sleep WAY better at night. This book is going to give you a 3-week program and after it's over I guarantee you will be a morning person, under the condition that you continue implementing what you've learned. First we will discuss how the book is laid out and then we will get right into it. I suggest that you read this book as it is intended; once you read the book layout and understand how the program works you should read the book one page per day. Each morning when you wake up you should immediately open the book to the proper day and follow the instructions. Good luck and lets mold you into a morning person so you can get the most out of your life!

Chapter 2: The Layout

For 3-weeks you are going to follow this book to a tee. If you waiver from the instructions in the book then you cannot expect it to work. It's really not hard to follow and with a little bit of motivation and discipline you should have no problem keeping up. I believe that reading something inspirational is the key to starting everyday, so at the beginning of each day there will be a quote to inspire you for the day ahead. After the quote there will be a short exercise activity that you must complete before eating breakfast. I know doing a quick workout isn't exactly the first thing you want to do when you get out of bed but trust me, it works wonders! By getting your body moving as soon as you wake up you're telling your body and mind that it's time to get the day started with a bang.

There will be a few different exercises that you will have to complete during the 3-week program so I will explain all of that now:

Understanding Workout Terminology:

When reading a workout the first number is the number of sets and the second number is the number of repetitions per set. So if you see 4 x 20, that means four sets of twenty reps per set. During a set you perform every exercise in order with no rest between exercises unless otherwise instructed. Some workouts will be timed such as 3 x 1:00, 1:00 off, 1:30 on. For this workout you would be doing each exercise in the set for one minute, resting for one minute and then doing that same exercise for one and a half minutes.

The Pushup:

Your stomach should be flat on the ground. Keep your arms at shoulder width apart, keep your back straight and make sure your chest touches the ground at the bottom and that your arms are straight at the end of every repetition.

The Burpee (Full):

Start in the standing position, jump down until your chest is on the ground, do a pushup keeping your back flat, jump your legs up into a squatted position and spring yourself up into the air with your arms reaching to the sky. With practice this movement will become fluid, but it remains a very challenging exercise.

The Burpee (Cardio):

Start in the standing position; jump down until you're in the push-up position with your arms straight ad legs straight. Don't do a push-up just jump your legs up into a squatted position and spring yourself up into the air with your arms reaching to the sky. With practice this movement will become fluid, but it remains a very challenging exercise.

The Squat:

Squats should be performed with your feet at shoulder width apart. Put your arms straight out in front of you and keep your back straight as you lower your bum to your ankles, keeping your legs parallel to one-another. Keep your back straight and keep your weight on your heels. Once you get as low as you can, use your legs to push yourself back up to the standing position, all the while keeping your back straight and your core tight

The Mountain Climber:

Mountain climbers are great for your core. To perform, hover above the ground keeping your body horizontal. You should be on your toes and hands with your arms straight. One at a time, bring your knees towards your chest in an alternating motion. Every time both legs go in and out, you have completed one repetition.

Leg Lifts:

For leg lifts you want to lie flat on your back with your legs completely straight. Bring your legs up from the ground until they are at 90 degrees relative to your torso and then lower them until they hover above the ground. During the exercise you can either have your hands on the floor, or under your bum if you're finding the exercise difficult.

Squat Jumps:

Squat jumps are performed just like a regular squat, but you jump into the air about 1 foot upon extension of the legs.

The Reverse Crunch:

Reverse crunches are performed by lying flat on your back with your hands on the ground beside you. Your legs should be bent with your feet on the ground and you simply bring your knees up towards your chest and then back down to perform one repetition.

The Russian Twist:

For a Russian twist, sit down, lean back and let your legs hover above the ground. Rotate your core around side to side with your hands in front of you and your chest up. Let your hands touch the ground on either side of you to complete one full rep.

The Plank:

 For a plank you want your stomach facing the ground. Put your elbows underneath your shoulders and lift yourself off the ground. Your weight should be on your elbows and your toes. Try to keep your back perfectly flat (don't sag your hips down to the ground or lift your bum really high into the air). Keep your abs tight and ensure that you have a comfortable base on your elbows/ forearms.

Leg Ins:

Leg ins are done from the plank position. Once in position, bring your right knee to your right elbow, and then back. Do the same with your left side and that equates to two reps.

Pikes:

 Pikes are also done from the plank position. Simply arch your back and stick your bum into the air, returning to the plank position to complete one repetition.

Flutter Kicks:

For flutter kicks you must lie on your back. Hover your legs above the ground and move them up and down as if you were kicking in the water. Up and down on each leg is one repetition.

U-Sits:

Sit on your bum with your knees bent and your feet hovering about one foot off the ground. The starting position for this exercise requires your legs to be straight (feet still hovering) and your arms should be straight, but off to the side as if you were trying to stop the walls from crushing in against you. To complete one repetition you must bend your knees up into your chest and clap your hands (arms remaining straight) in front of your knees.

The Lunge Walk:

One leg at a time, step one foot out in front of you as far as you can, while dropping the opposite knee down to the ground (don't actually touch the knee on the ground, but get as close as you can). Get a nice smooth walking pattern going as you continue to switch legs.

The Sit-Up With Twist:

Keep your feet flat on the ground, knees pointed up to the sky and your hands touching your ears. Once you have fully sat up I want you to touch your right elbow to your left knee and then your left elbow to your right knee. This gets your abs a little more involved than a regular sit-up does.

Wall Sits:

Put your back flat against a wall, bend your legs at about 90 degrees and hover above the ground like you are sitting in an invisible chair. Hold the position for as long as the specified time says.

Chapter 3: The Program

WEEK 1, DAY 1:

The secret of getting ahead is getting started.

- Mark Twain

By procrastinating and not taking action, you will always fail! Today's workout isn't going to be too hard, I want you to do the exercises slowly and ensure that you are using proper technique as described in the previous chapter. Remember to do these morning workouts as soon as you turn your alarm clock off. Try to attack the workouts with high intensity. Today's workout is:

2 sets of:

3 burpees (full)

30 seconds rest

20 mountain climbers

30 seconds rest

10 squats

30 seconds rest

*Rest 2 minutes between sets.

WEEK 1, DAY 2:

I have no idols; I admire work, dedication and competence.

- Aryton Senna

Not attempting to achieve your goals is as grave a sin as any. For today's workout you're going to go for a short walk. Don't waste any time, just hop out of bed, put on some appropriate workout clothing, grab your shoes and head out the door (or jump onto the treadmill if you have access to one).

4 sets of:

Walk for 2 minutes, jog for 1 minute

* Don't rest between sets. I suggest doing two sets out and two sets back so that you finish where you started. If time allows you could do all four sets out and then just walk back to where you started.

WEEK 1, DAY 3:

Patience, persistence and perspiration make and unbeatable combination for success.

- Napoleon Hill

Remember the above quote as the 3 P's. If you lack any of the P's you're sure to fail at whatever you're trying to do in life. This workout is going to be an ab burner!

Perform 3 sets of:

20 leg lifts

5 push-ups

10 reverse crunches

30-second plank

30-second wall sit

*Rest 10 seconds between exercises and 1-minute between sets.

WEEK 1, DAY 4:

The journey of a thousand miles must begin with a single step.

- Lao Tzu

Remember to keep your goals in focus, but never become overwhelmed by the size of those goals. Take things day by day and eventually you will end up where you want to be. Even people who have achieved seemingly impossible goals had to break them down into extremely small steps and tackle those steps on a daily basis. This workout will test your endurance.

Complete as many repetitions of each exercise as you can in 10 minutes:

2 burpees (cardio)

4 push-ups

6 squats

8 lunge walks

10 u-sits

*No rest. Go down the list of exercises continuously until the 10 minutes is up.

WEEK 1, DAY 5:

Somebody should tell us, right at the start of our lives, that we are dying. Whatever you want to do, do it now. There are only so many tomorrows.

-Michael Landen

Live your life as if it were fleeting, but then keep in mind that it truly is fleeting. Work everyday to become the person you truly want to be. This workout will force you to prove to yourself how badly you want to achieve your goals.

For 10 minutes repeat the following set:

- Plank for as long as you can, once you cannot plank anymore, perform 10 burpees (full).

- Wall sit for as long as you can, once you cannot wall sit anymore, perform 10 burpees (cardio).

*There is no rest during this workout. You are simply planking until you fail, doing 10 burpees and then wall sitting until you fail and doing 10 burpees. You are to do this continuously for 10 minutes.

WEEK 1, DAY 6:

The ladder of success is never crowded at the top.

-Napoleon Hill

Most people settle for mediocrity, which means there are many people striving to be average, but very few striving to be great. You want to fall into the latter category. Get your legs ready for a tough workout!

Complete 4 sets of the following:

15 squats

20 lunge walks

20 mountain climbers

10 squat jumps

*Rest 20 seconds between exercises and 1 minute between sets.

WEEK 1, DAY 7:

The most difficult thing is the decision to act, the rest is merely tenacity.

-Amelia Earhart

Making the conscious decision to act can be very hard to do, but not for you; you've already completed a full week of the program, congratulations! Don't stop now, keep up the hard work and don't waiver from the program at all.

Perform 2 sets of the following exercises:

10 push-ups

20 squats

30 mountain climbers

40 flutter kicks

1-minute plank

*Rest for 15 seconds between exercises and 2 minutes between sets.

WEEK 2, DAY 1:

All people dream, but not equally.

- T.E. Lawrence

As I mentioned earlier, most people strive for mediocrity because they don't believe that their dreams are realistic. If your dream is to lose 40 pounds but you make your goal to lose only 20 pounds, you are, whether intentionally or not, lacking belief in your own abilities and desire. Never sell yourself short; if you don't dream big you make it impossible to achieve big things. Once you settle even one time in your life you open the floodgates to a lifetime of average achievements.

Perform 3 sets of the following for a total of 12 minutes of work:

- Walk for 1 minute

- Jog for 1 minute

- Run fast for 1 minute

*No Rest. Use the 1-minute of walking to recover for the next 2 minutes of jogging and fast running.

WEEK 2, DAY 2:

And so you touch this limit, something happens and you suddenly can go a little bit further. With your mind power, your determination, your instinct, and the experience as well, you can fly very high.

-Aryton Senna

Limits are merely figments of people's imaginations. You won't truly know your limits until you push, stretch and surpass them, at which point you will then know that you have higher limits. Life should be a continuation of this cycle; if you do this you will become a very empowered person. Today's workout is designed to test your limits and get you sweating!

In 12 minutes complete as many sets of the following exercises as you possibly can:

- 10 push-ups

- 10 sit-ups with twist

- 10 squat jumps

*Rest as you need but remember that you're trying to complete as many sets as you can in 12 minutes.

WEEK 2, DAY 3:

I'd rather live in regret of failure than in regret of never trying.

- MJ Demarco

When your life starts winding to an end you will likely have more regrets about the things you didn't do than about the things you did do. Personally, I don't to be an old man in a Lazy Boy recliner beating myself up over all of the things I never did in my life. Today's workout is going to be tough, but if you don't do it you will regret it!

Perform 1 set of the following:

50 flutter kicks

1-minute plank

30 mountain climbers

20 burpees (cardio)

25 u-sits

20 pikes

20 push-ups

15 leg ins

2-minute wall sit

*Rest as little as possible between exercises. Try to go from one exercise to another with as little transition time as possible.

WEEK 2, DAY 4:

Always do your best, what you plant now you will harvest later.

- O.G. Mandino

The harder you work now the more it will payoff later. Very few people enjoy waking up and immediately doing a quick workout, but then again very few people are happy with their fitness and productivity levels. You must pay a price to have what you want in life. Do your best in this workout and see how many reps you can do of every exercise.

Complete as many reps as you can of every exercise. Once you complete as many reps as you can, rest for 2 minutes and move on to the next exercise.

- Burpees (cardio)

- Plank (For time)

- Squats

- Flutter kicks

- Push-ups

*Rest for 2 minutes between exercises.

WEEK 2, DAY 5:

You can do anything you set your mind to.

-Marshall Mathers (Eminem)

Your mind is a powerful tool. If you become obsessed with success and achieving goals your mind will find a way to make your dreams a reality. This requires more than just a positive mindset though; it will take blood, sweat, tears and perhaps even years.

Complete one set of the following:

5 push-ups

5 squat jumps

4 push-ups

4 squat jumps

3 push-ups

3 squat jumps

2 push-ups

2 squat jumps

1 push-up

1 squat jump

2 push-ups

2 squat jumps

3 push-ups

3 squat jumps

4 push-ups

4 squat jumps

5 push-ups

5 squat jumps

* Rest 15 seconds between each push-up/ squat jump set. For example: at the start of the workout you would do 5 push-ups and 5 squat jumps with no rest in between, but then after you complete 5 reps of each you would rest for 15 seconds before completing 4 push-ups and 4 squat jumps.

WEEK 2, DAY 6:

The starting point of all achievement is a strong, burning desire.

-Napoleon Hill

A strong desire doesn't mean just wanting something, it means fully dedicating yourself to something. If you strongly desire to lose weight and become a more productive person you must dedicate yourself to this desire. If you've made it this far in the book then you're doing a good job and you've gotten in the habit of working out. Developing good habits is one of the hardest parts of adopting a healthier lifestyle.

Complete 2 sets of the following:

Jog for 5 minutes

20 Russian twists

20 mountain climbers

5 burpees (full)

* Rest for 2 minutes between sets and don't rest between exercises.

WEEK 2, DAY 7:

It in your moments of decision that your destiny is shaped.

- Tony Robbins

Life is made up of millions of tiny day-to-day decisions. Make enough small positive decisions and your life will gradually transform in a positive way, but do the opposite and your life will slowly (perhaps even too slow for you to notice) take a turn for the worst.

Perform 3 sets of the following:

10 squats

9 leg lifts

8 push-ups

7 pikes

6 lunge walks

5 sit-ups with twist

4 squat jumps

3 burpees (full)

2 reverse crunches

1-minute plank

*Rest two minutes between sets. Rest a maximum of 10 seconds between exercises.

WEEK 3, DAY 1:

The person at the top of the mountain didn't fall there.

- Vince Lombardi

Getting results and being successful never happens by mistake!
This is the final week of the program so let's get it started. Today's
workout is short, but don't let it fool you, it's meant to be intense.
Get it done as fast as possible.

Complete 4 sets of the following:

10 burpees (cardio)

20 reverse crunches

30 mountain climbers

*No rest!

WEEK 3, DAY 2:

Normal is not something to aspire to it's something to get away from.

- Jodie Foster

If you're striving to be normal then you are saying that you want to be like everyone else. News flash: most people aren't happy with their lives, most people wish they were doing something else for a job, most people aren't healthy and most people aren't who you should aspire to be. Today's workout may be a little out of the ordinary and you may have never done one like it, but trust me, it's a full body blast!

Perform 2 sets of the following exercises. Perform each exercise for 40 seconds and then rest for 20 seconds before moving to the next exercise:

- Burpees (full)

- Squat jumps

- Plank

- Pikes

- Mountain climbers

- Lunge walks

- Flutter kicks

- Push-ups

* No rest except for the 20 seconds between exercises.

WEEK 3, DAY 3:

Kites rise highest against the wind, not with it.

- Winston Churchill

On your path to achieving your goals you will certainly be met with resistance. Sometimes this resistance serves the purpose of showing you how badly you truly want something. Anything worth achieving is not going to be easy to do, or else everyone would already be doing it.

Perform 3 sets of the following:

2 minute jog

30 squats

20 lunge walks

10 squat jumps

*Rest only 2 minutes between sets.

WEEK 3, DAY 4:

There's no difference between a pessimist who says, "Oh it's hopeless, so don't bother doing anything," and an optimist who says, "don't bother doing anything, it's going to turn out fine anyway." Either way, nothing happens.

- Yvon Chouinard

Talk is cheap and for some people, talking is all they ever do. Taking action requires planning and persistence while talking only requires a mouth and an idea. The former leads to success while the latter only leads to more talking, normally in the form of excuses.

Complete 2 sets of the following exercises. On the first set do 20 seconds of each exercise and rest for 40 seconds between exercises. On the second set do thirty seconds of each exercise and rest for 1 minute between sets.

- Pikes

- Push-ups

- Sit-ups with twist

- Burpees (full)

- Mountain climbers

- Squats

WEEK 3, DAY 5:

If everything seems under control, you're not going fast enough.

- Mario Andretti

If you're constantly comfortable in your life then you aren't challenging yourself enough. If you aren't being challenged then you are unable to learn and grow as a human being. Take time every single day to challenge yourself or you will become weak and complacent.

Complete 3 sets of 20 reps of the following exercises:

- Leg lifts

- Burpees (cardio)

- Pikes

- Push-ups

- Russian twists

*Rest 2 minutes between sets and 20 seconds between exercises.

WEEK 3, DAY 6:

Great achievement is usually born of great sacrifice, and is never the result of selfishness.

- Napoleon Hill

Sacrificing an extra 20 minutes of sleep to complete these workouts is what you must do if you want to lose weight, boost productivity and live a healthier life.

In 12 minutes complete as many sets as you can of the following:

10 push-ups

10 mountain climbers

10 burpees (cardio)

* Rest as you need but remember you're trying to complete as many sets as possible.

WEEK 3, DAY 7:

Because in a split second, it's gone.

- Aryton Senna

The above is one of my favorite quotes from the Formula 1 racing legend himself. While the context of the quote was Senna's attempt at describing the opportunity to pass other drivers, the quote is memorable because Senna died when his car malfunctioned and crashed into a wall. He went from being the champion of the world to a mere memory in less than a second. Life is precious and time is a limited commodity. Don't waste a single second.

Complete 5 sets of the following exercises:

30 Russian twists

25 push-ups

30 flutter kicks

25 jumping jacks

10 burpees (cardio)

*Rest 10 seconds between exercises and 1 minute between sets.

Conclusion:

Congratulations on completing this program. Working out in the morning can be difficult in the beginning, but once you get in the routine I think you'll find it's the best way to go. I hope this book has helped you boost your productivity level and wake you up in the morning! Once you complete this program you can change and alter the workouts to your liking and make your own program and continue with longer and more difficult workouts.

It has become my life's mission to enhance the lives of others by helping them get fit and healthy. Keep your eyes open for my newest books as I am constantly creating and publishing new material. I am also in the process of starting an online coaching company where I personally coach and guide you to achieve your fitness goals. The coaching that I will offer will allow me to personally speak with you (via skype) and create a personalized program for you that will help you reach your goals. If you have any questions about this book or the program feel free to email me at johnmayo@hotmail.com.

Thanks for reading and happy training!

If you enjoyed this book I'm sure you will like some of my other titles. Check out this sample:

How To Get Abs: 2-in-1 Flat Stomach Boxed Set

How to Get Abs Fast With An Extensive 6-Week Workout Plan

John Mayo

© 2015

Table of Contents:

1) Introduction:

If you don't have to work hard for something, then it's usually not worth getting!

   We all know why you're here, so let's get right down to it. First things first, congratulations for taking it upon yourself to flatten out your stomach. Abs and a flat stomach are probably the most desired aspect of the human body for a lot of people. Human beings will put themselves through immense pain at the gym, just so they can feel good about themselves when they take off their shirts. Can you really blame these people though? Let's face it; abs and a flat stomach look great and it's completely understandable that people want to achieve this look.

   So who am I and why should you care? I'm the guy who's going to help you achieve your fitness goals. I'm a guy who has had abs for almost his entire life. I'm not being cocky about it; it's just a fact. I have been an athlete for my entire life and fitness is something that I take very seriously. I am a kayaking coach in Nova Scotia, Canada, and my passion is helping people increase their fitness level. Since abs are a very sought after thing, I really enjoy helping people flatten their stomachs and get ripped abs.

   Let me be honest though, abs are not easy to get, nor are they easy to maintain. Anything in life that is worthwhile takes hard work and dedication to achieve and getting abs is no different. I have a theory about abs; I think that one of the main things that make abs so sexy is that when people see a flat stomach or ripped abs, they understand the hard work and self-discipline associated with this achievement. I think a lot of people view a person's stomach as a direct reflection of their personality, so when somebody has no belly fat, people generally think of that person as dedicated, focused and determined. Unless of course they cheated and got liposuction. Perhaps you think this theory is a stretch, but I believe it to hold quite true for most people.

   So what makes this fitness book different from all the other "get abs fast" books out there? One word, honesty. I will not lie to you and tell you that at the end of this 6-week program you will have the chiseled abs and flat stomach that you've always desired. But if you take the information, workout techniques and fitness strategies that I am going to provide to you in the following pages, apply them continuously and never give up, you will undoubtedly get the results that you desire.

Make no mistake; this is going to be a difficult task. I talk a lot in my other fitness books about forming good habits. One you make something a habit, it becomes automatic and easy. The less you have to think about making good, healthy choices, the better off your life will be. This is why it is very important to get into good fitness routines and stick with them! That's where I come in. I am very good at getting people into healthy routines and creating manageable programs that will better their health. This specific book is obviously going to focus on how to get abs and if you follow along and do not stray from my program, I can almost guarantee that you will see results. Strap yourselves in, focus, tighten those abs up and let's get going!

2) Abs Behind the Scenes:

If you're going to ignore your eating habits completely and strictly focus on exercise, don't bother reading any further. Contrary to popular belief, diet is the MOST important factor for getting abs. It doesn't matter how many fantastic abdominal exercises you do everyday, if you're eating fatty, deep fried, over-processed foods, you're not going to see results.

-What I Try to Avoid:

Fried foods, white rice, bread, potatoes, cereal, beer/ liquid carbs, fatty sauces, trans fats (obviously), high fructose corn syrup (glucose- fructose in Canada).

* I consume every single thing listed above; I just try to consume very minimal amounts of each.

-What I Typically Try to Eat:

Quinoa & quinoa pasta, whole grain or multigrain bread (if I eat bread at all), avocadoes, kale, spinach, max 2-3 eggs a day, brown rice, ground flaxseed (frozen or refrigerated), chia seeds (great mixed with water), chicken breast, ground tomatoes (substitute for pasta sauce), bananas, natural peanut/ almond butter, dates, unsalted nuts and almonds, black beans, cliff bars, mixed vegetables, unsweetened almond milk, unsweetened coconut water/ oil, LOTS AND LOTS OF WATER!

If you only allow healthy food in your living space, it will make things a lot easier when you have a craving for something bad. Here are some meals you could make that I really enjoy: